The Patient's Guide

Uterine Fibroid Embolization

Adam E. M. Eltorai, MD, PhD
Matthew Czar Taon, MD, RPVI, WCC
Terrance T. Healey, MD

Praeclarus Press, LLC

www.PraeclarusPress.com

Praeclarus Press, LLC
2504 Sweetgum Lane
Amarillo, Texas 79124 USA
806-367-9950
www.PraeclarusPress.com

DISCLAIMER
The information contained in this publication is advisory only and is not intended to replace sound clinical judgment or individualized patient care. The author disclaims all warranties, whether expressed or implied, including any warranty as the quality, accuracy, safety, or suitability of this information for any particular purpose.

ISBN: 9781946665294
©2020 Matthew Czar Taon. All rights reserved.
Email: matthew.taon@gmail.com

Cover Design: Ken Tackett
Developmental Editing: Kathleen Kendall-Tackett
Copy Editing: Chris Tackett
Layout & Design: Nelly Murariu

CONTENTS

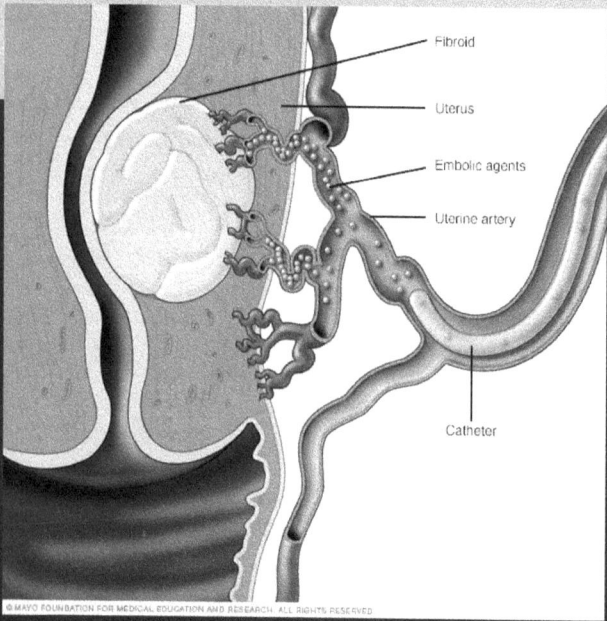

Fibroid

Uterus

Embolic agents

Uterine artery

Catheter

WHAT IS UTERINE FIBROID EMBOLIZATION (UFE)? WHAT IS UTERINE ARTERY EMBOLIZATION (UAE)?

The word embolization is derived from the Greek word *"embolos,"* which means "to plug." **Uterine fibroid embolization** is a minimally invasive treatment in which the arterial blood flow supplying uterine fibroids is plugged/blocked. In patients who are experiencing pain, excessive bleeding, or symptoms due to the bulkiness of their fibroids, such as abdominal distension, pelvic pressure, constipation, pain with intercourse, or frequent urination, uterine fibroid embolization is an effective method of treating these symptoms.

This minimally invasive technique of accessing the uterine arteries and blocking them is not only limited to treating uterine fibroids. In fact, it can be used to stop severe pelvic bleeding caused by trauma, malignant gynecological tumors, or hemorrhage after childbirth. A more general term for this technique is called **uterine artery embolization**.

In a uterine fibroid or uterine artery embolization procedure, an interventional radiologist, a physician specialized in image-guided procedures, uses live X-ray imaging, called fluoroscopy, to guide a thin, flexible tube, called a catheter, through an artery in the wrist or groin into the arteries supplying the uterine fibroids. Small particles are then injected into the uterine arteries to block their blood flow and cause the fibroids to shrink. The procedure is safe and extremely effective at relieving symptoms associated with fibroids.

Uterine fibroid embolization does not require general anesthesia. Rather, it is performed under local anesthesia and **conscious sedation**, a type of sedation in which the patient is awake and able to tolerate procedures while maintaining his or her own cardiorespiratory function.

After the procedure, patients generally stay at the hospital overnight and can return home the next day.

Why is a uterine fibroid embolization performed?

Patients with uterine fibroids may experience pain, excessive bleeding, or symptoms due to the bulkiness of their fibroids such as abdominal distension, pelvic pressure, constipation, pain with intercourse, or frequent urination. Uterine fibroid embolization is performed as a minimally invasive procedure to alleviate these symptoms. In fact, up to 90% of patients demonstrate long-term symptom control.

Uterine artery embolization is one method of treating uterine fibroids. Other surgical treatment options include myomectomy, which is surgical removal of a fibroid while leaving the remainder of the uterus in-tact, and hysterectomy, which is complete surgical removal of the uterus. There are also medical treatment options that may directly address bleeding symptoms or may try to shrink uterine fibroids by addressing the hormonal components associated with fibroids.

An additional minimally invasive procedure is magnetic resonance-guided focused ultrasound ablation. This utilizes focused ultrasound beams to ablate and destroy fibroids. This technique is promising but demonstrates a relatively higher rate of reintervention.

The decision to undergo uterine fibroid embolization should not be made in isolation. Rather, it should be a collaborative decision made among a patient, an interventional radiologist, and a gynecologist. An interventional radiologist will see a patient in the clinic and review her history, symptoms, age, prior fibroid therapies, preference regarding uterine sparing therapy, desire for future pregnancy, risks for the procedure, and ultimately make a clinical recommendation as to whether she is a candidate for uterine artery embolization.

HOW DO I PREPARE FOR MY FIBROID EMBOLIZATION?

During the evaluation, whether a patient is a candidate for uterine fibroid embolization, patients usually undergo imaging of the uterus by magnetic resonance imaging (MRI) or ultrasound. This allows a thorough evaluation of the size, number, and location of the patient's fibroids.

Prior to your procedure, you should report to your doctor all medications that you are taking, including herbal supplements, and if you have any allergies, especially to local anesthetic medications, general anesthesia, or to contrast materials containing iodine.

Women should always inform their physician and X-ray technologist if there is any possibility that they are pregnant.

It is recommended that you do not eat or drink anything after midnight before your procedure. Your doctor will tell you which of your medications you may take in the morning.

You should plan to stay overnight at the hospital following your procedure and should plan for transportation back home upon safe discharge from the hospital.

WHAT IS THE EQUIPMENT LIKE?

Your interventional radiologist may use various imaging devices to perform the procedure. An ultrasound machine may be used to visualize arteries in your wrist or groin to gain access into your arterial system. A live X-ray machine, called a **fluoroscope**, converts X-rays into video images and is used to guide the procedure.

The patient lies on a radiographic table during the procedure and will usually have an intravenous (IV) line place for medication administration. The patient will be draped to ensure a sterile, clean procedure.

A thin, long tube called a catheter will be used to traverse through your arteries into the arteries feeding the uterus and fibroids.

There are various materials used to block the arteries feeding the fibroids; these are called embolic agents. A few **embolic agents** include microspheres, tiny spheres of various sizes that may be made of polyacrylamide; polyvinyl alcohol, a finely-ground plastic material; and Gelfoam, a gelatin sponge material.

Throughout the duration of the procedure, your blood pressure and vitals will be monitored with various devices to ensure that you are safe.

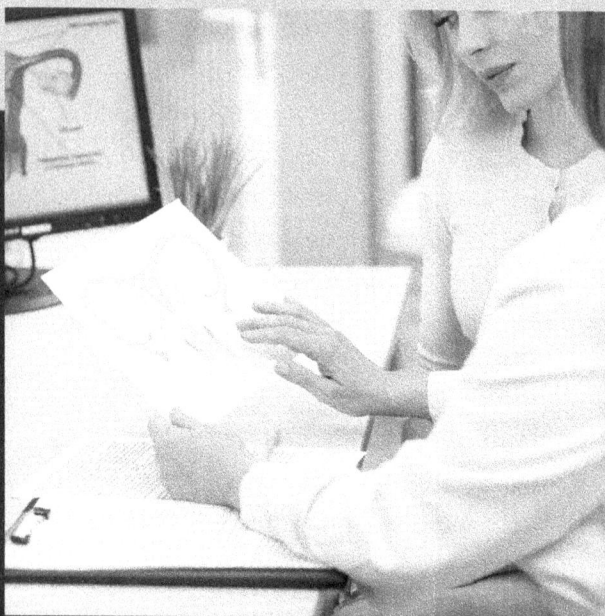

WHAT DOES THE PROCEDURE INVOLVE?

The goal of uterine fibroid embolization is to block the arteries supplying blood flow to fibroids, causing them the fibroids to shrink, thereby alleviating the patient's fibroid-related symptoms. The procedure is typically performed in a fluoroscopy suite or in an operating room. You will be positioned on an examination table and will be connected to monitors that track your heart rate, blood pressure, and pulse during the procedure. A nurse or technologist will insert an intravenous (IV) line into a vein in your hand or arm so that sedative medications can be given intravenously. The area of your body where the catheter is to be inserted, usually the wrist or the groin, will be sterilized and covered with a surgical drape. Your physician will then numb the area with a local anesthetic.

A very small skin incision is made at the access site. Using ultrasound and/or X-ray guidance, a thin, long catheter is inserted into your radial artery in your wrist or your femoral artery in the groin area.

A contrast agent will be injected to provide a roadmap of your arteries to guide the positioning of the catheter into your uterine arteries. Once the catheter is in position, the embolic agents are released into both the right and left uterine arteries. At the end of the procedure, the catheter will be removed, and pressure will be applied to stop any bleeding. The procedural site is then covered with a dressing. Most patients are observed in the hospital overnight and will receive anti-inflammatory medications and analgesic medication to alleviate any post-procedural pain. Procedural times vary, but the procedure is usually completed within 60- 90 minutes.

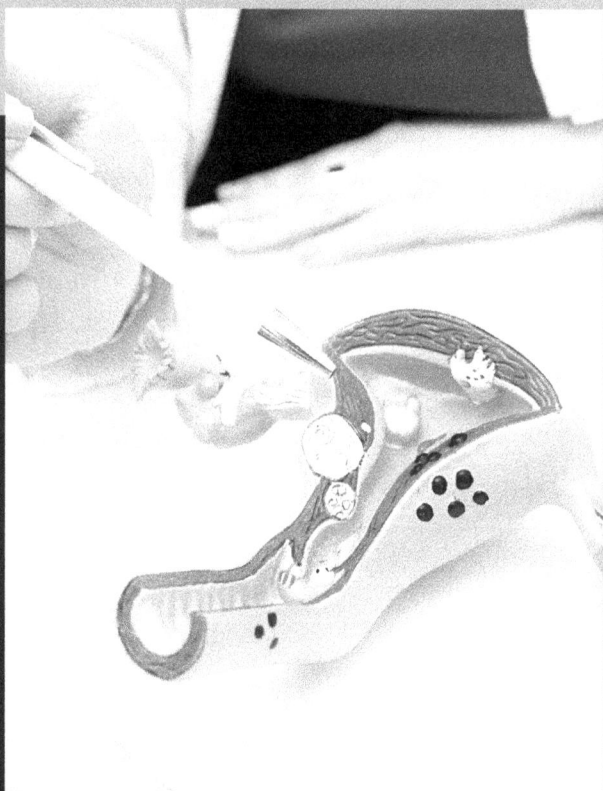

WHAT DOES A UTERINE FIBROID EMBOLIZATION FEEL LIKE?

You will be lying on your back on a procedural table for the entirety of the procedure. Monitors will be placed to monitor your heart rate and blood pressure. You may feel a cold sensation as the nurse or technologist is cleaning the procedural site. You will feel a slight pinprick when the nurse or technologist is obtaining intravenous (IV) access. You will feel relaxed, drowsy, and comfortable once the sedation medication is administered intravenously. You will feel a slight word when the local anesthetic is injected into the procedural site. You may feel pressure at the access site in your wrist or groin when the catheter is inserted into the vein or artery. When contrast is being injected into your body, you may experience a warm feeling which dissipates rapidly. While you are in the hospital, your pain will be controlled with a narcotic. In some settings, you may be provided with a hand-held button that allows you to administered pain medication when necessary; this is called patient-controlled analgesia. Patients usually stay in the hospital overnight after the procedure and are able to return home the next day. You may experience pelvic cramps, nausea, and a low-grade fever for several days after the procedure. Generally, the cramps are most severe during the first 24 hours after the procedure. This highlights the importance of immediate post-procedural pain control. The cramps will improve rapidly over the next several days and, upon safe discharge home, the discomfort is usually tolerated with oral pain medication. Patients are usually able to return to their normal activities within one to two weeks after the procedure.

In terms of symptoms, menstrual bleeding is expected to markedly decrease during the first cycle and gradually increase to a new level that is usually greatly improved when compared to pre-procedural bleeding. **Bulk-related symptoms** take approximately 6 weeks to be noticeable, and over a period of months, the fibroids to continue to shrink and soften.

What happens after the procedure?

After the procedure is done, you will be admitted to the hospital overnight and administered anti-inflammatory medications and narcotic pain medication. After an overnight hospital stay, you should be able to return home the next day.

You may experience pelvic cramps, nausea, and low-grade fever for several days after the procedure. These symptoms are usually worse within the first 24 hours after the procedure but subside rapidly in the following days. Upon safe discharge home, you will be given medications for pain but should be able to return to your normal activities within one to two weeks.

How will I know the results of my procedure?

Your interventional radiologist will be able to tell you immediately how the procedure went. However, it will take time to see the true outcome of the procedure. The expected outcomes following uterine fibroid embolization include 50%-60% fibroid size reduction, 40%-50% uterine size reduction, 88%-92% reduction of bulk symptoms, greater than 90% elimination of abnormal uterine bleeding, and 80%-90% patient satisfaction (Dariushnia, et al., 2014). Generally, bleeding symptoms are noticeably reduced by the next menstrual cycle, whereas bulk symptoms become noticeable after approximately 6 weeks.

WHAT ARE THE RISKS AND BENEFITS OF A UTERINE FIBROID EMBOLIZATION?

Risks:

⚠ General risks with any catheter-based procedure include pain, infection, bleeding, and injury to adjacent structures.

⚠ Risks more specific to uterine fibroid embolization include fibroid expulsion requiring dilatation and curettage, early menopause, failed procedure requiring a hysterectomy, and infertility.

⚠ Since iodinated contrast may be used during the procedure, there is a risk that an adverse allergic reaction may occur. The symptoms may range from mild itching to severe shortness of breath.

⚠ Since fluoroscopy utilizes X-rays to provide imaging, there are radiation exposure risks.

Benefits:

✓ Uterine fibroid embolization is a minimally invasive procedure that does not require open or laparoscopic surgery.

✓ Recovery time for uterine fibroid embolization is much shorter compared to myomectomy and hysterectomy, and patients are able to return to their usual daily activities much sooner.

✓ The expected outcomes following uterine fibroid embolization include 50%-60% fibroid size reduction, 40%-50% uterine size reduction, 88%-92% reduction of bulk symptoms, greater than 90% elimination of abnormal uterine bleeding, and 80%-90% patient satisfaction.

ARE THERE LIMITATIONS TO A UTERINE FIBROID EMBOLIZATION?

U terine fibroid embolization should only be performed in women who are symptomatic from their fibroids. It should not be performed in the setting of active pelvic inflammation or infection. It should not be performed in patients who are currently pregnant. A woman with an allergy or prior adverse reaction to iodine-based contrast materials should obtain pretreatment with steroids before undergoing uterine fibroid embolization or should consider a different treatment option.

FREQUENTLY ASKED QUESTIONS

Q: Does a uterine fibroid embolization involve any radiation?

A: Yes. Fluoroscopy is a technique in which live X-rays guide an interventional radiologist to treat a patient's fibroids. Since X-rays are used, there is radiation exposure.

Q: Are there any risks to a uterine fibroid embolization?

A: Yes. General risks with any catheter-based procedure include pain, infection, bleeding, and injury to adjacent structures. Risks more specific to uterine fibroid embolization include fibroid expulsion requiring dilatation and curettage, early menopause, failed procedure requiring a hysterectomy, and infertility.

Q: How long will my uterine fibroid embolization procedure take?

A: It varies based on the complexity of the anatomy but usually 60-90 minutes.

Q: When will my results be available?

A: Your interventional radiologist will be able to tell you how the procedure went immediately after the procedure is complete.

GLOSSARY

UTERINE FIBROID EMBOLIZATION

A minimally invasive treatment in which the arterial blood flow supplying uterine fibroids is plugged/blocked.

UTERINE ARTERY EMBOLIZATION

A more general term for the minimally invasive technique of blocking arterial blood flow to the uterus. The differences in the naming of the procedure highlights the fact that this procedure is not only limited to treating fibroids but can also be used to treat severe pelvic bleeding.

EMBOLIC AGENTS

Material used to block the blood vessels. These may be composed of various microspheres, plastic-type materials, or gelatin sponge material.

CONSCIOUS SEDATION

A type of sedation in which the patient is awake and able to tolerate procedures while maintaining his or her own cardiorespiratory function.

FLUOROSCOPY

Live X-ray imaging that converts X-rays into video images used to guide minimally invasive procedures.

BULK-RELATED FIBROID SYMPTOMS

Abdominal distension, pelvic pressure, constipation, pain with intercourse, or frequent urination.

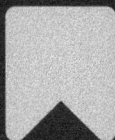

ADDITIONAL RESOURCES

Society of Interventional Radiology
Patient Center:
https://www.sirweb.org/patients/uterine-fibroids/

Radiologyinfo.org
https://www.radiologyinfo.org/en/info.cfm?pg=ufe

American College of Obstetricians
and Gynecologists
https://www.acog.org/-/media/For-Patients/
faq074.pdf

MY CONTACTS

NAME

CONTACT

NAME

CONTACT

NAME

CONTACT

NAME

CONTACT

MY APPOINTMENTS

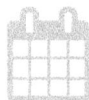

MONDAY

Date:
_____

THURSDAY

Date:
_____

TUESDAY

Date:
_____

FRIDAY

Date:
_____

WEDNESDAY

Date:
_____

SATURDAY

Date:
_____

MY QUESTIONS

MY QUESTIONS

MY QUESTIONS

MY QUESTIONS

MY QUESTIONS

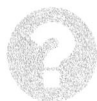

MY NOTES

MY NOTES

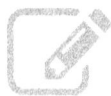

MY NOTES

MY NOTES

MY NOTES

MY NOTES

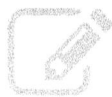

www.ingramcontent.com/pod-product-compliance
Lightning Source LLC
Chambersburg PA
CBHW071423200326

41520CB00014B/3547